Pescatarian Diet Made Easy

Loose Weight & Gain Health with Tasty Fish, Seafood and Vegetable Dishes

Jacob Aiello

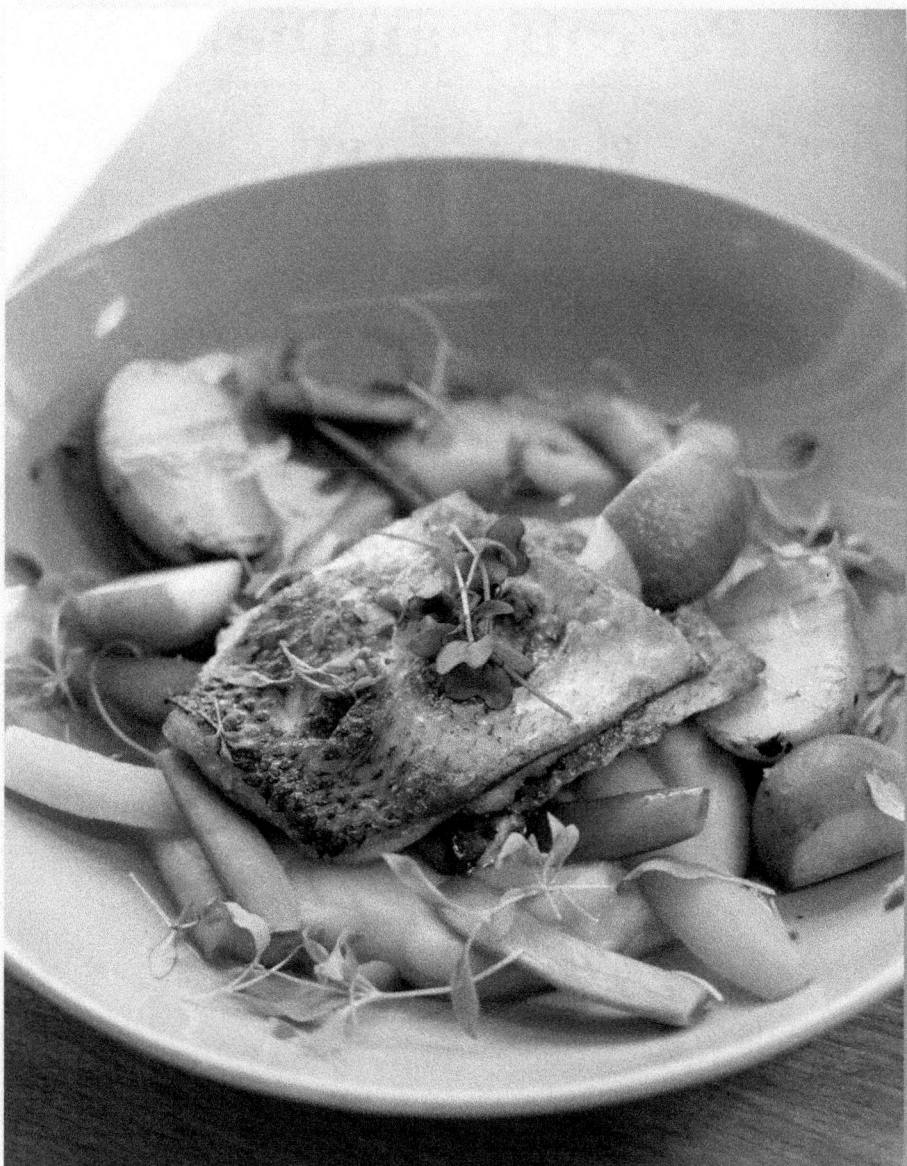

Table of Contents

Simple Mahi Mahi

Preparation Time: 10 minutes

Cooking Time: 12 minutes

Serve: 4

Nutritional Value (Amount per Serving):

- Calories 361
- Fat 30.7 g
- Carbohydrates 0 g
- Sugar 0 g
- Protein 21.3 g
- Cholesterol 121 mg
- **Ingredients:**
- 4 mahi-mahi fillets
- 2/3 cup butter
- Pepper
- Salt

Directions:

1. Preheat the air fryer to 350 F.
2. Season Mahi-mahi fillets with pepper and salt.
3. Place fish fillets into the air fryer basket and cook for 12 minutes.
4. Add butter into the pan and melt over medium heat.
5. Pour melted butter over fish fillets and serve.

Pesto Mahi Mahi

Preparation Time: 10 minutes

Cooking Time: 15 minutes

Serve: 2

Nutritional Value (Amount per Serving):

- Calories 92
- Fat 0.1 g
- Carbohydrates 0.3 g
- Sugar 0 g
- Protein 21.3 g
- Cholesterol 40 mg

Ingredients:

- 2 mahi-mahi fillets
- 3/4 cup basil pesto
- Pepper
- Salt

Directions:

1. Preheat the air fryer to 300 F.
2. Season fish fillets with pepper and salt.
3. Place fish fillets into the air fryer basket. Top fish with basil pesto and cook for 12-15 minutes.
4. Serve and enjoy.

Easy Lemon Dill Fish Fillets

Preparation Time: 10 minutes

Cooking Time: 14 minutes

Serve: 2

Nutritional Value (Amount per Serving):

- Calories 156
- Fat 7.1 g
- Carbohydrates 1.1 g
- Sugar 0.2 g
- Protein 21.4 g
- Cholesterol 40 mg

Ingredients:

- 2 mahi-mahi fillets
- 1 tbsp dill, chopped
- 2 lemon sliced
- 1 tbsp olive oil

- 1 tbsp lemon juice
- Pepper
- Salt

Directions:

1. In a small bowl, mix olive oil and lemon juice.
2. Season fish fillets with pepper and salt and brush with oil mixture.
3. Place fish fillets into the air fryer basket and top with dill and lemon slices and cook at 400 F for 12-14 minutes.
4. Serve and enjoy.

Delicious Tuna Patties

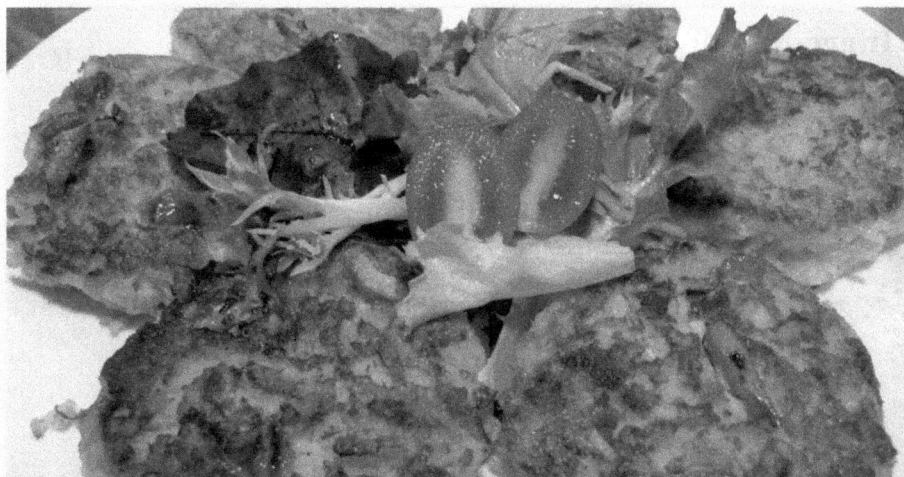

Preparation Time: 10 minutes

Cooking Time: 10 minutes

Serve: 5

Nutritional Value (Amount per Serving):

- Calories 128
- Fat 2.5 g
- Carbohydrates 0.9 g
- Sugar 0.5 g

- Protein 24.1 g
- Cholesterol 91 mg

Ingredients:

- 2 eggs, lightly beaten
- 15 oz can tuna, drained
- 1/2 tsp dried herbs
- 1/2 tsp garlic powder
- 2 tbsp onion, minced
- 1 celery stalk, chopped
- 3 tbsp parmesan cheese, grated
- 1/2 cup whole-wheat breadcrumbs
- 1 tbsp lemon juice
- 1 lemon zest
- Pepper
- Salt

Directions:

1. Add all ingredients into the bowl and mix until well combined.
2. Make equal shape of patties from mixture and place onto the parchment-lined baking sheet. Place patties in the refrigerator for 1 hour.

3. Spray air fryer basket with cooking spray.

4. Place patties into the air fryer basket and cook at 360 F for 10 minutes. Flip patties halfway through.

5. Serve and enjoy.

Cheesy Tuna Patties

Preparation Time: 10 minutes

Cooking Time: 10 minutes

Serve: 4

Nutritional Value (Amount per Serving):

- Calories 167
- Fat 8.4 g
- Carbohydrates 6.2 g
- Sugar 0.9 g
- Protein 16.3 g
- Cholesterol 65 mg

Ingredients:

- 1 egg
  - oz tuna, drained
- 1/2 tsp onion powder
- 1/2 tsp garlic powder

- 1 tsp paprika
- 2 tbsp hot sauce
- 1 oz cheddar cheese, shredded
- 1 oz parmesan cheese, shredded
- 1/4 cup breadcrumbs
- Pepper
- Salt

Directions:

1. Add all ingredients into the bowl and mix until well combined.
2. Spray air fryer basket with cooking spray.
3. Make patties from the mixture and place into the air fryer basket and cook at 400 F for 10 minutes.
4. Serve and enjoy.

Tasty Tuna Steaks

Preparation Time: 10 minutes

Cooking Time: 10 minutes

Serve: 2

Nutritional Value (Amount per Serving):

- Calories 683
- Fat 46.4 g
- Carbohydrates 4.6 g
- Sugar 1.1 g
- Protein 61.2 g
- Cholesterol 70 mg

Ingredients:

- 1 lb tuna
- 1 tbsp garlic, minced
- 4 tbsp olive oil
- 1 tbsp garlic powder

- 1/2 tsp thyme
- Pepper
- Salt

Directions:

1. In a bowl, mix oil, garlic, garlic powder, thyme, pepper, and salt. Add tuna steaks and mix well and place in the refrigerator for 15 minutes.

2. Place tuna steaks into the air fryer basket and cook at 400 F for 10 minutes.

3. Serve and enjoy.

Flavorful Tuna Patties

Preparation Time: 10 minutes

Cooking Time: 10 minutes

Serve: 8

Nutritional Value (Amount per Serving):

- Calories 88
- Fat 3.6 g
- Carbohydrates 2.2 g
- Sugar 0.8 g
- Protein 11.3 g
- Cholesterol 57 mg

Ingredients:

- 2 eggs
- 10 oz can tuna, chopped
- 2 tbsp mayonnaise
- 1/2 tsp garlic powder

- 1/4 cup fresh mint, chopped
- 1/4 cup feta cheese, crumbled
- 1/2 onion, chopped
- Pepper
- Salt

Directions:

1. Add all ingredients into the bowl and mix until well combined.
2. spray air fryer basket with cooking spray.
3. Make patties from the mixture and place into the air fryer basket and cook at 400 F for 10 minutes.
4. Serve and enjoy.

BBQ Salmon

Preparation Time: 10 minutes

Cooking Time: 25 minutes

Serve: 4

Nutritional Value (Amount per Serving):

- Calories 323
- Fat 11.2 g
- Carbohydrates 22 g
- Sugar 20.3 g
- Protein 35.8 g
- Cholesterol 78 mg

Ingredients:

- 4 salmon fillets

For sauce:

- 2 tsp soy sauce
- 3 tbsp balsamic vinegar
- 3 tbsp brown sugar
- 1 cup tomato ketchup
- Pepper
- Salt

Directions:

1. Add all sauce ingredients into the small saucepan and bring to boil over medium heat. Turn heat to low and simmer for 15 minutes.
2. Spray salmon fillets with cooking spray and season with pepper and salt.
3. Place salmon fillets into the air fryer basket and cook at 380 for 5 minutes.
4. Brush salmon fillets with BBQ sauce and cook for 5 minutes more.
5. Serve and enjoy.

Crispy Coconut Shrimp

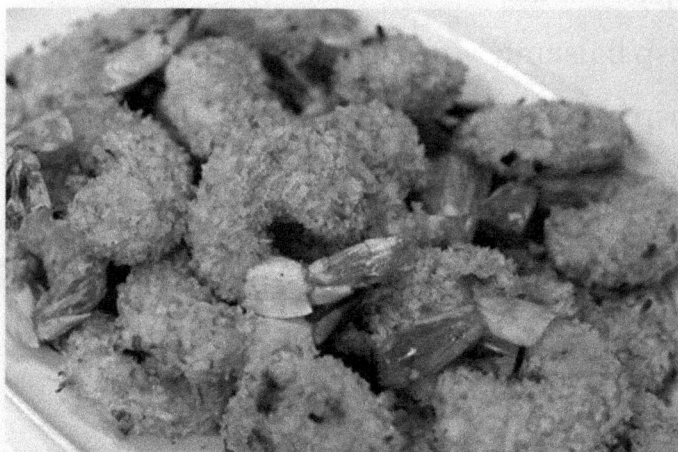

Preparation Time: 10 minutes

Cooking Time: 5 minutes

Serve: 4

Nutritional Value (Amount per Serving):

- Calories 184

- Fat 6.5 g

- Carbohydrates 19.1 g

- Sugar 1.3 g

- Protein 11.9 g
- Cholesterol 140 mg

Ingredients:

- 2 eggs, lightly beaten
- 20 large shrimp, peeled
- 1/4 cup whole-wheat breadcrumbs
- 1/2 cup shredded coconut
- 1/4 tsp garlic powder
- 1/2 cup all-purpose flour
- Pepper
- Salt

Directions:

1. in a small bowl, add eggs and whisk well.
2. In a shallow dish, mix breadcrumbs, shredded coconut, garlic powder, flour, pepper, and salt.
3. Preheat the air fryer to 400 F.
4. Dip shrimp in egg then coat with breadcrumb mixture.
5. Spray air fryer basket with cooking spray.

6. Place shrimp into the air fryer basket and cook for 5 minutes.
7. Serve and enjoy.

Tasty Shrimp Fajitas

Preparation Time: 10 minutes

Cooking Time: 9 minutes

Serve: 4

Nutritional Value (Amount per Serving):

- Calories 206
- Fat 5.7 g
- Carbohydrates 11.3 g
- Sugar 5.2 g
- Protein 26.9 g
- Cholesterol 239 mg

Ingredients:

- 1 lb shrimp, thawed
- 3/4 tbsp Fajita seasoning
- 1 tbsp olive oil
- 1 small onion, sliced

- 3 small bell peppers, sliced
- Pepper
- Salt

Directions:

1. Preheat the air fryer to 375 F.
2. Add shrimp and remaining ingredients into the bowl and toss well.
3. Add shrimp mixture into the air fryer basket and cook for 9 minutes. Stir halfway through.
4. Serve and enjoy.

Garlic Honey Shrimp

Preparation Time: 10 minutes

Cooking Time: 10 minutes

Serve: 6

Nutritional Value (Amount per Serving):

- Calories 229
- Fat 1.5 g
- Carbohydrates 35.1 g
- Sugar 24.7 g
- Protein 19.8 g
- Cholesterol 159 mg

Ingredients:

- 16 oz shrimp, peeled & deveined
- 16 oz mixed vegetables
- 2 tbsp cornstarch
- 1 tsp ginger garlic paste

- 2 tbsp ketchup
- 1/2 cup soy sauce
- 1/2 cup honey

Directions:

1. Add soy sauce, ketchup, ginger garlic paste, and honey into the small saucepan and cook over medium heat until warm.
2. Add cornstarch and stir constantly until thickened.
3. Remove saucepan from heat. Pour sauce over shrimp and vegetables and toss well.
4. Preheat the air fryer to 350 F.
5. Spray air fryer basket with cooking spray.
6. Add shrimp and vegetables into the air fryer basket and cook for 10 minutes.
7. Serve and enjoy.

Delicious Fish Bites

Preparation Time: 10 minutes

Cooking Time: 10 minutes

Serve: 4

Nutritional Value (Amount per Serving):

- Calories 234
- Fat 2 g
- Carbohydrates 37.7 g
- Sugar 0.2 g
- Protein 16.4 g
- Cholesterol 61 mg

Ingredients:

- 1 egg, lightly beaten
- 1 lb cod fillets, cut into 1-inch strips
- 1/2 tsp lemon pepper seasoning
- 1/2 tsp smoked paprika

- 1/2 cup whole-wheat breadcrumbs
- 1/2 cup all-purpose flour
- Pepper
- Salt

Directions:

1. In a small bowl, add egg and whisk well.
2. In a separate bowl, mix flour, pepper, and salt.
3. In a shallow dish, mix breadcrumbs, paprika, and lemon pepper seasoning.
4. Coat fish strips with flour then dip in egg and finally coat with breadcrumb mixture.
5. Preheat the air fryer to 400 F.
6. Spray air fryer basket with cooking spray.
7. Place coated fish strips into the air fryer basket and cook for 10 minutes. Turn fish strips halfway through.
8. Serve and enjoy.

Garlic Cheese Shrimp

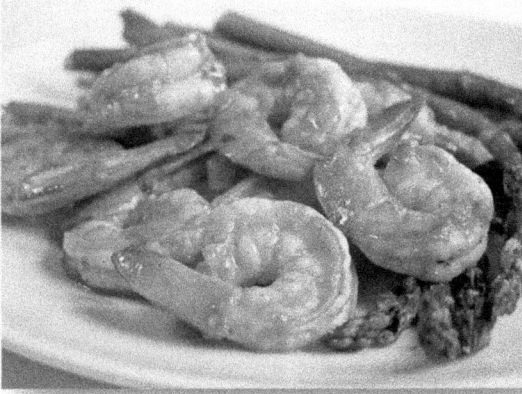

Preparation Time: 10 minutes

Cooking Time: 8 minutes

Serve: 6

Nutritional Value (Amount per Serving):

- Calories 223
- Fat 7.3 g
- Carbohydrates 3.1 g
- Sugar 0.1 g
- Protein 34.6 g

- Cholesterol 318 mg

Ingredients:

- 2 lbs cooked shrimp, peeled & deveined
- 2 tbsp olive oil
- 3/4 tsp onion powder
- 1 tsp basil
- 1/2 tsp oregano
- 2/3 cup parmesan cheese, grated
- 1 tbsp garlic, minced
- Pepper
- Salt

Directions:

1. Add shrimp and remaining ingredients into the bowl and toss until well coated.
2. Add shrimp into the air fryer basket and cook at 350 F for 8 minutes.
3. Serve and enjoy.

Crispy Shrimp Popcorn

Preparation Time: 10 minutes

Cooking Time: 5 minutes

Serve: 4

Nutritional Value (Amount per Serving):

- Calories 356
- Fat 9.6 g
- Carbohydrates 27.6 g
- Sugar 0.2 g
- Protein 37.9 g
- Cholesterol 331 mg

Ingredients:

- 2 eggs, lightly beaten
- 5 oz oat flour
- 2 oz parmesan cheese, grated
- 8 oz whole-wheat breadcrumbs

- 1 lb shrimp, cooked & peeled
- Pepper
- Salt

Directions:

1. In a small bowl, add eggs and whisk well.
2. In a separate bowl, add oat flour.
3. In a shallow dish, mix breadcrumbs, cheese, pepper, and salt.
4. Coat shrimp with oat flour then dip in eggs and finally coat with breadcrumb mixture.
5. Place coated shrimp into the air fryer basket and cook at 400 F for 5 minutes.
6. Serve and enjoy.

Lemon Garlic Shrimp

Preparation Time: 10 minutes

Cooking Time: 8 minutes

Serve: 4

Nutritional Value (Amount per Serving):

- Calories 161
- Fat 4.8 g
- Carbohydrates 1.9 g
- Sugar 0 g
- Protein 25.9 g
- Cholesterol 246 mg

Ingredients:

- 1 lb shrimp, peeled & deveined
- 2 tbsp parmesan cheese, grated
- 1/2 tsp garlic, minced
- 1 tsp lemon juice

- 1 tbsp butter, melted
- Salt

Directions:

1. Add shrimp and remaining ingredients into the bowl and toss well.
2. Add shrimp mixture into the air fryer basket and cook at 400 F for 8 minutes.
3. Serve and enjoy.

Shrimp Boil

Preparation Time: 10 minutes

Cooking Time: 12 minutes

Serve: 4

Nutritional Value (Amount per Serving):

- Calories 221
- Fat 14.8 g
- Carbohydrates 1.1 g
- Sugar 0.2 g
- Protein 19.4 g
- Cholesterol 131 mg

Ingredients:

- 6 oz shrimp, peeled & deveined
- 1 tbsp old bay seasoning
- 2 tbsp onion, diced
- 2 mini corn on the cobs

- 2 cups baby potatoes, boiled & halved
- 7 oz smoked sausage, sliced

Directions:

1. Add shrimp and remaining ingredients into the bowl and toss well.
2. Add shrimp mixture into the air fryer basket and cook for 12 minutes. Mix halfway through.
3. Stir well and serve.

Crispy Salt & Pepper Shrimp

Preparation Time: 10 minutes

Cooking Time: 10 minutes

Serve: 4

Nutritional Value (Amount per Serving):

- Calories 228
- Fat 9.1 g
- Carbohydrates 9.3 g
- Sugar 1 g
- Protein 26.4 g
- Cholesterol 239 mg

Ingredients:

- 1 lb shrimp
- 2 tbsp olive oil
- 3 tbsp rice flour
- 1 tsp sugar, crushed

- 2 tsp ground pepper
- Salt

Directions:

1. Add shrimp, oil, rice flour, sugar, pepper, and salt into the bowl and toss well.
2. Spray air fryer basket with cooking spray.
3. Add shrimp into the air fryer basket and cook at 325 F for 10 minutes.
4. Serve and enjoy.

Asian Shrimp

Preparation Time: 10 minutes

Cooking Time: 6 minutes

Serve: 4

Nutritional Value (Amount per Serving):

- Calories 214
- Fat 9 g
- Carbohydrates 6 g
- Sugar 3.2 g
- Protein 26.4 g
- Cholesterol 239 mg

Ingredients:

- 1 lb shrimp, peeled & deveined
- For marinade:
- 1 tbsp lemon juice
- 1 tsp garlic, minced

- 1/8 tsp cayenne
- 1 tbsp maple syrup
- 2 tbsp soy sauce
- 2 tbsp olive oil
- Pepper
- Salt

Directions:

1. Add shrimp and marinade ingredients into the bowl and mix well and place in the refrigerator for 15 minutes.
2. Spray air fryer basket with cooking spray.
3. Place shrimp into the air fryer basket and cook at 400 F for 6 minutes.
4. Serve and enjoy.

Flavorful Blackened Shrimp

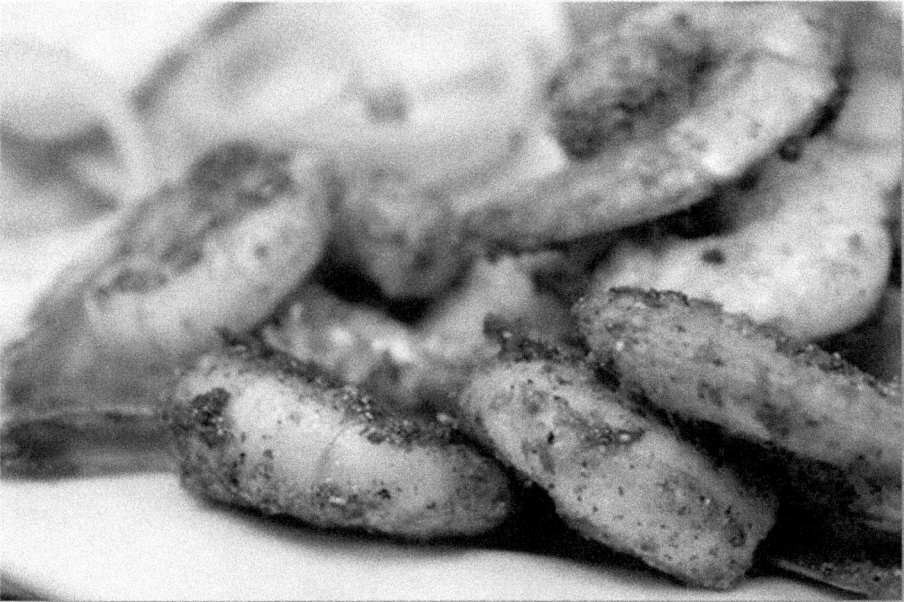

Preparation Time: 10 minutes

Cooking Time: 10 minutes

Serve: 4

Nutritional Value (Amount per Serving):

- Calories 204

- Fat 9.1 g

- Carbohydrates 3.6 g
- Sugar 0.5 g
- Protein 26.2 g
- Cholesterol 239 mg

Ingredients:

- 1 lb shrimp, peeled & deveined
- 2 tsp smoked paprika
- 1/4 tsp cayenne
- 1 tsp dried oregano
- 1 tsp garlic powder
- 1 tsp onion powder
- 2 tbsp olive oil
- Pepper
- Salt

Directions:

1. Add shrimp and remaining ingredients into the bowl and toss well.
2. Preheat the air fryer to 400 F.

3. Spray air fryer basket with cooking spray.

4. Add shrimp into the air fryer basket and cook for 8-10 minutes or until cooked through.

5. Serve and enjoy.

Shrimp Dinner

Preparation Time: 10 minutes

Cooking Time: 8 minutes

Serve: 4

Nutritional Value (Amount per Serving):

- Calories 364
- Fat 21.2 g
- Carbohydrates 7.3 g
- Sugar 3.2 g
- Protein 35.6 g
- Cholesterol 275 mg

Ingredients:

- 1 lb shrimp, peeled
- 2 tbsp olive oil
- 1 bell pepper, cut into 1-inch pieces
- 1 squash, cut into slices

- 1 zucchini, cut into slices
- 6 oz sausage, sliced
- 1 tbsp Cajun seasoning
- Salt

Directions:

1. Preheat the air fryer to 400 F.
2. Add shrimp and remaining ingredients into the bowl and toss well.
3. Add shrimp mixture into the air fryer basket and cook for 8 minutes.
4. Serve and enjoy.

Shrimp with Veggie

Preparation Time: 10 minutes

Cooking Time: 15 minutes

Serve: 4

Nutritional Value (Amount per Serving):

- Calories 196
- Fat 6.6 g
- Carbohydrates 6.7 g
- Sugar 2.7 g
- Protein 26.9 g
- Cholesterol 241 mg

Ingredients:

- 1 lb shrimp, peeled & deveined
- 1/4 cup parmesan cheese, grated
- 1 tbsp Italian seasoning
- 1 tbsp garlic, minced

- 1 tbsp olive oil

- 1 bell pepper, chopped

- 1 zucchini, chopped

- Pepper

- Salt

Directions:

1. Add shrimp and remaining ingredients into the bowl and toss well.

2. Add shrimp mixture into the air fryer basket and cook at 390 F for 15 minutes. Stir halfway through.

3. Serve and enjoy.

Perfect Shrimp Skewers

Preparation Time: 10 minutes

Cooking Time: 8 minutes

Serve: 4

Nutritional Value (Amount per Serving):

- Calories 70
- Fat 1.1 g
- Carbohydrates 1.3 g
- Sugar 0 g
- Protein 13 g
- Cholesterol 119 mg

Ingredients:

- 1/2 lb shrimp, peeled & deveined
- 1 tbsp cilantro, chopped
- 1 lemon juice
- 1/2 tsp ground cumin

- 1/2 tsp smoked paprika
- 1/2 tsp garlic paste
- Salt

Directions:

1. Add shrimp and remaining ingredients into the bowl and mix well. Cover and place in the refrigerator for 15 minutes.
2. Thread shrimp onto the soaked skewers.
3. Preheat the air fryer to 350 F.
4. Place shrimp skewers into the air fryer basket and cook for 8 minutes.
5. Serve and enjoy.

Shrimp with Onion & Pepper

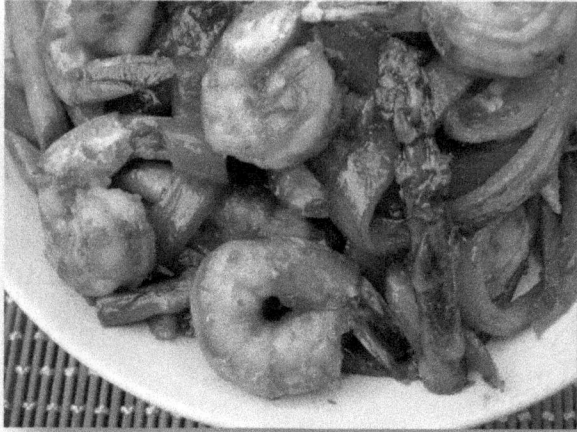

Preparation Time: 10 minutes

Cooking Time: 15 minutes

Serve: 4

Nutritional Value (Amount per Serving):

- Calories 183
- Fat 5.6 g
- Carbohydrates 5.9 g
- Sugar 2.2 g

- Protein 26.4 g
- Cholesterol 239 mg

Ingredients:

- 1 lb shrimp, peeled & deveined
- 1/8 tsp cayenne
- 1/2 tsp garlic powder
- 1 tsp chili powder
- 1 tbsp olive oil
- 1/2 onion, cut into chunks
- 1 bell pepper, cut into chunks
- Pepper
- Salt

Directions:

1. Add shrimp and remaining ingredients into the bowl and toss well.
2. Add shrimp mixture into the air fryer basket and cook at 330 F for 15 minutes. Stir halfway through.
3. Serve and enjoy.

Hawaiian Shrimp

Preparation Time: 10 minutes

Cooking Time: 8 minutes

Serve: 4

Nutritional Value (Amount per Serving):

- Calories 257
- Fat 13.5 g
- Carbohydrates 6.5 g
- Sugar 0.1 g
- Protein 26.2 g
- Cholesterol 269 mg

Ingredients:

- 1 lb shrimp
- 1 1/2 tsp paprika
- 2 tbsp cornstarch
- 1 tbsp garlic, minced

- 1/4 cup butter
- Pepper
- Salt

Directions:

1. Add shrimp, cornstarch, paprika, pepper, and salt into the bowl and toss until well coated.
2. Spray air fryer basket with cooking spray.
3. Add shrimp into the air fryer basket and cook at 350 F for 8 minutes.
4. Melt butter in a pan over medium heat, once butter is melted then add garlic and sauté for 30 seconds.
5. Pour garlic butter mixture over shrimp and serve.

Lemon Old Bay Shrimp

Preparation Time: 10 minutes

Cooking Time: 10 minutes

Serve: 4

Nutritional Value (Amount per Serving):

- Calories 148
- Fat 3.4 g
- Carbohydrates 1.9 g
- Sugar 0 g
- Protein 25.9 g
- Cholesterol 243 mg

Ingredients:

- 1 lb shrimp, peeled & deveined
- 1 tbsp old bay seasoning
- 1/2 tsp garlic, minced
- 1/2 tsp lemon juice

- 1/2 tbsp butter, melted
- Pepper
- Salt

Directions:

1. Add shrimp and remaining ingredients into the bowl and toss well.
2. Add shrimp mixture into the air fryer basket and cook at 390 F for 8-10 minutes. Stir halfway through.
3. Serve and enjoy.

Southwest Shrimp

Preparation Time: 10 minutes

Cooking Time: 6 minutes

Serve: 4

Nutritional Value (Amount per Serving):

- Calories 143
- Fat 2.9 g
- Carbohydrates 1.7 g
- Sugar 0 g
- Protein 25.8 g
- Cholesterol 241 mg

Ingredients:

- 1 lb shrimp, peeled & deveined
- 1 1/2 tsp southwestern seasoning
- 1 tsp butter, melted

Directions:

1. In a bowl, toss shrimp with seasoning and melted butter.
2. Preheat the air fryer to 400 F.
3. Add shrimp into the air fryer basket and cook for 6 minutes.
4. Serve and enjoy.

Easy Spicy Shrimp

Preparation Time: 10 minutes

Cooking Time: 7 minutes

Serve: 4

Nutritional Value (Amount per Serving):

- Calories 150
- Fat 3.4 g
- Carbohydrates 2.7 g
- Sugar 0.1 g
- Protein 26.1 g
- Cholesterol 239 mg

Ingredients:

- 1 lb shrimp
- 1/4 tsp ground mustard
- 1/4 tsp ground cumin
- 1/4 tsp oregano

- 1/4 tsp thyme

- 1/4 tsp cayenne

- 1/4 tsp garlic powder

- 1/2 tsp paprika

- 1 tsp chili powder

- 1 tsp olive oil

- Pepper

- Salt

Directions:

1. Preheat the air fryer to 400 F.
2. Add shrimp and remaining ingredients into the bowl and toss well.
3. Add shrimp mixture into the air fryer basket and cook for 7 minutes. Stir halfway through.
4. Serve and enjoy.

Perfect Air Fried Shrimp

Preparation Time: 10 minutes

Cooking Time: 8 minutes

Serve: 4

Nutritional Value (Amount per Serving):

- Calories 158
- Fat 4.4 g
- Carbohydrates 2.1 g
- Sugar 0.2 g
- Protein 25.9 g
- Cholesterol 239 mg

Ingredients:

- 1 lb shrimp
- 1/2 tsp Italian seasoning
- 1/4 tsp paprika
- 1/2 tsp garlic powder

- 2 tsp olive oil
- Pepper
- Salt

Directions:

1. Preheat the air fryer to 400 F.
2. Add shrimp and remaining ingredients into the bowl and toss well.
3. Add shrimp mixture into the air fryer basket and cook for 8 minutes.
4. Serve and enjoy.

Healthy Cod Fish Fillets

Preparation Time: 10 minutes

Cooking Time: 10 minutes

Serve: 4

Nutritional Value (Amount per Serving):

- Calories 64
- Fat 2.3 g
- Carbohydrates 7 g
- Sugar 0.4 g
- Protein 3.8 g
- Cholesterol 82 mg

Ingredients:

- 2 eggs
- 1 tsp garlic powder
- 1 tsp lemon pepper seasoning
- 1 cup parmesan cheese, grated

- 1 cup almond flour
- 1/2 cup whole-wheat breadcrumbs
- 1/4 cup all-purpose flour
- 4 cod fillets
- Pepper
- Salt

Directions:

1. In a small bowl, whisk eggs with pepper and salt.
2. In a shallow dish, mix breadcrumbs, almond flour, cheese, lemon pepper seasoning, and garlic powder.
3. In a separate bowl, add flour.
4. Coat fish fillets with flour then dip in the egg mixture and finally coat with breadcrumb mixture.
5. Place coated fish fillets into the air fryer basket and cook at 350 F for 8-10 minutes.
6. Serve and enjoy.

Flavorful Salmon Steak

Preparation Time: 10 minutes

Cooking Time: 14 minutes

Serve: 2

Nutritional Value (Amount per Serving):

- Calories 441
- Fat 34.1 g
- Carbohydrates 0.5 g
- Sugar 0 g
- Protein 34.9 g
- Cholesterol 140 mg

Ingredients:

- 2 salmon steaks
- 2 tsp ground sage
- 4 tbsp butter, melted

- Pepper
- Salt

Directions:

1. In a small bowl, mix butter, sage, pepper, and salt.
2. Brush salmon steaks with butter mixture and place into the air fryer basket and cook at 400 F for 14 minutes.
3. Serve and enjoy.

Honey Garlic Shrimp Skewers

Preparation Time: 10 minutes

Cooking Time: 5 minutes

Serve: 4

Nutritional Value (Amount per Serving):

- Calories 332
- Fat 8.9 g
- Carbohydrates 38 g
- Sugar 35 g
- Protein 26.8 g
- Cholesterol 239 mg

Ingredients:

- 1 lb shrimp
- 2 tsp garlic, minced
- 2 tbsp olive oil

- 3 tbsp soy sauce
- 1/2 cup honey

Directions:

1. Add shrimp, garlic, oil, soy sauce, and honey into the bowl and mix well. Cover and place in the refrigerator for overnight.
2. Thread marinated shrimp onto the soaked wooden skewers.
3. Place shrimp skewers into the air fryer basket and cook at 400 F for 5 minutes.
4. Serve and enjoy.

Flavorful Spicy Shrimp

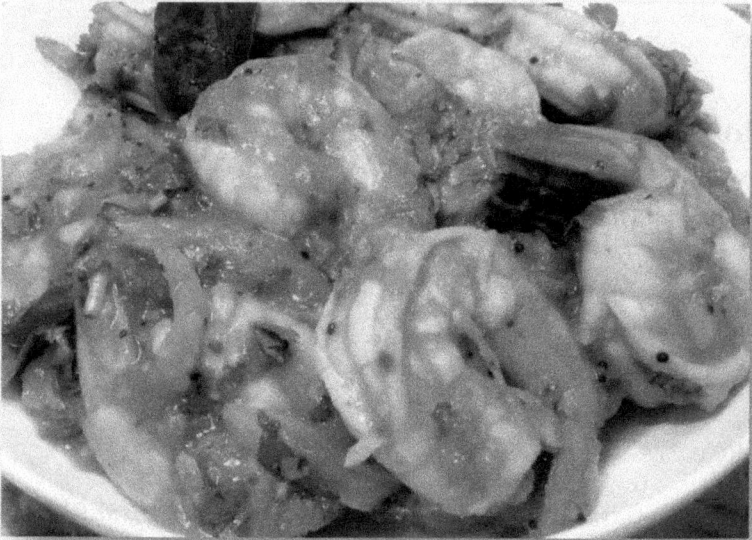

Preparation Time: 10 minutes

Cooking Time: 10 minutes

Serve: 4

Nutritional Value (Amount per Serving):

- Calories 287
- Fat 4.2 g
- Carbohydrates 6.6 g

- Sugar 1.5 g
- Protein 52.6 g
- Cholesterol 478 mg

Ingredients:

- 2 lb shrimp, peeled & deveined
- 1 tbsp lemon juice
- 2 tbsp soy sauce
- 1 tsp garlic powder
- 1 tsp sugar
- 1 tsp ground cumin
- 1 tsp liquid smoke
- 1 tsp chili powder
- 1 tbsp Tabasco sauce
- 1 tsp paprika
- Pepper
- Salt

Directions:

1. Add shrimp and remaining ingredients into the bowl and toss well.
2. Add shrimp mixture into the air fryer basket and cook at 400 F for 10 minutes. Stir halfway through.
3. Serve and enjoy.

Scallops with Sauce

Preparation Time: 10 minutes

Cooking Time: 7 minutes

Serve: 4

Nutritional Value (Amount per Serving):

- Calories 238
- Fat 15 g
- Carbohydrates 4.5 g
- Sugar 1 g
- Protein 20.9 g
- Cholesterol 57 mg

Ingredients:

- 1 lb sea scallops
- 2 tsp garlic, minced
- 3 tbsp heavy cream
- 1/4 cup pesto

- 1 tbsp olive oil
- Pepper
- Salt

Directions:

1. Season scallops with pepper and salt.
2. Place scallops into the air fryer basket and cook at 320 F for 5 minutes.
3. In a pan, add cream, pesto, oil, and garlic and cook for 2 minutes.
4. Pour sauce over cooked scallops and serve.

Tasty Tuna Cakes

Preparation Time: 10 minutes

Cooking Time: 6 minutes

Serve: 4

Nutritional Value (Amount per Serving):

- Calories 113
- Fat 2.7 g
- Carbohydrates 5.9 g
- Sugar 0.7 g
- Protein 15.6 g
- Cholesterol 56 mg

Ingredients:

- 1 egg
- 7 oz can tuna
- 1/4 cup whole-wheat breadcrumbs
- 1 tbsp mustard

- Pepper
- Salt

Directions:

1. Add all ingredients into the bowl and mix until well combined.
2. Make patties from the mixture and place into the air fryer basket and cook at 400 F for 6 minutes. Turn patties halfway through.
3. Serve and enjoy.

Easy Salmon Patties

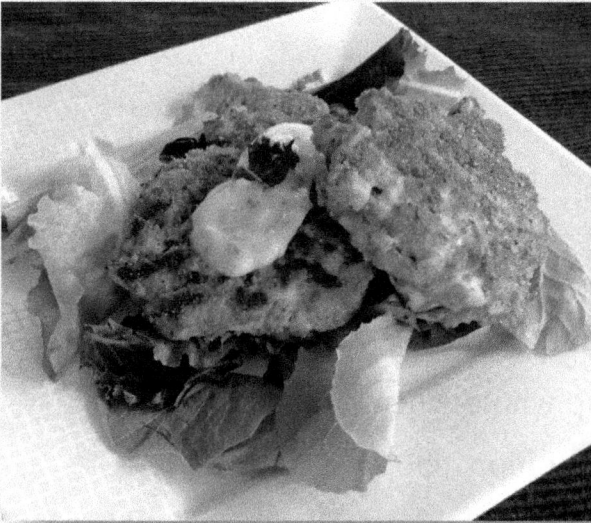

Preparation Time: 10 minutes

Cooking Time: 10 minutes

Serve: 4

Nutritional Value (Amount per Serving):

- Calories 157
- Fat 7.1 g
- Carbohydrates 0.9 g

- Sugar 0.4 g
- Protein 21.1 g
- Cholesterol 95 mg

Ingredients:

- 1 egg
- 1 tsp dill weed
- 1/2 cup whole-wheat breadcrumbs
- 1/4 cup onion, chopped
- 14 oz can salmon, remove bones & skin
- Pepper
- Salt

Directions:

1. Add all ingredients into the bowl and mix until well combined.
2. Make patties from the mixture and place into the air fryer basket and cook at 370 F for 10 minutes. Turn patties halfway through.
3. Serve and enjoy.

Quick & Easy Scallops

Preparation Time: 10 minutes

Cooking Time: 4 minutes

Serve: 2

Nutritional Value (Amount per Serving):

- Calories 126
- Fat 3.2 g
- Carbohydrates 2.9 g
- Sugar 0 g
- Protein 20.2 g
- Cholesterol 40 mg

Ingredients:

- 8 scallops
- 1 tsp olive oil
- Pepper
- Salt

Directions:

1. Preheat the air fryer to 390 F.
2. Add scallops, oil, pepper, and salt into the bowl and toss well.
3. Add scallops into the air fryer basket and cook for 4 minutes. Turn scallops halfway through.
4. Serve and enjoy.

Cajun Scallops

Preparation Time: 10 minutes

Cooking Time: 6 minutes

Serve: 2

Nutritional Value (Amount per Serving):

- Calories 99
- Fat 3 g
- Carbohydrates 2.1 g
- Sugar 0 g
- Protein 15.1 g
- Cholesterol 30 mg

Ingredients:

- 6 scallops
- 1/2 tsp Cajun seasoning
- 1 tsp olive oil
- Salt

Directions:

1. Preheat the air fryer to 400 F.
2. Add scallops, oil, Cajun seasoning, and salt into the bowl and toss well.
3. Add scallops into the air fryer basket and cook for 6 minutes. Turn scallops halfway through.
4. Serve and enjoy.

Creamy Scallops

Preparation Time: 10 minutes

Cooking Time: 10 minutes

Serve: 4

Nutritional Value (Amount per Serving):

- Calories 220
- Fat 13.7 g
- Carbohydrates 3.4 g
- Sugar 0.1 g
- Protein 19.4 g
- Cholesterol 76 mg

Ingredients:

- 1 lb sea scallops
- 1 tbsp white wine
- 1 tsp garlic, minced
- 2 tsp lemon juice

- 3 tbsp heavy cream
- 3 tbsp butter
- Pepper
- Salt

Directions:

1. Preheat the air fryer to 400 F.
2. Season scallops with pepper and salt and place into the air fryer basket and cook for 10 minutes. Turn scallops halfway through.
3. Melt butter in a pan over medium heat.
4. Add garlic and sauté for 30 seconds. Add wine, lemon juice, and heavy cream and stir until thickened.
5. Pour sauce over cooked scallops and serve.

Flavors Crab Cakes

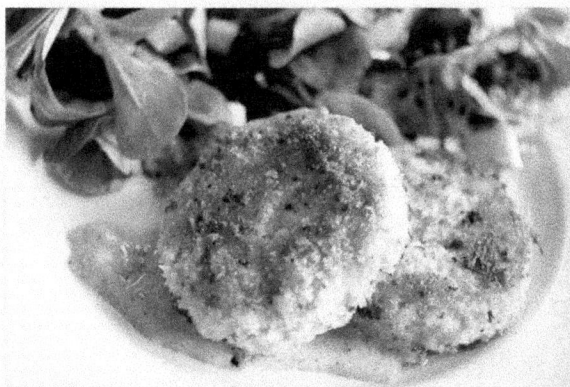

Preparation Time: 10 minutes

Cooking Time: 12 minutes

Serve: 4

Nutritional Value (Amount per Serving):

- Calories 187
- Fat 8.3 g
- Carbohydrates 8 g
- Sugar 2.1 g
- Protein 16.5 g
- Cholesterol 105 mg

Ingredients:

- 1 egg
- 1 lb crab meat
- 1 tbsp capers
- 1 roasted red pepper, diced
- 2 green onions, chopped
- 2/3 cup whole-wheat breadcrumbs
- 1 tbsp parsley, chopped
- 1/2 lemon juice
- 2 tsp old bay seasoning
- 1 tbsp soy sauce
- 1 tbsp Dijon mustard
- 1/4 cup mayonnaise
- Salt

Directions:

1. Preheat the air fryer to 360 F.
2. Spray air fryer basket with cooking spray.
3. Add all ingredients into the mixing bowl and mix until well combined.

4. Make the equal shape of patties from the mixture and place into the air fryer basket and cook for 7 minutes.
5. Flip patties and cook for 5 minutes more.
6. Serve and enjoy.

Quick & Easy Salmon Patties

Preparation Time: 10 minutes

Cooking Time: 8 minutes

Serve: 6

Nutritional Value (Amount per Serving):

- Calories 105
- Fat 4.8 g
- Carbohydrates 0.6 g
- Sugar 0.2 g
- Protein 14.2 g
- Cholesterol 64 mg

Ingredients:

- 1 egg
- 1 tsp paprika
- 2 green onions, minced

- 2 tbsp fresh coriander, chopped
- 14 oz can salmon, drain & remove bones Salt

Directions:

1. Preheat the air fryer to 360 F.
2. Add all ingredients into the mixing bowl and mix until well combined.
3. Make the equal shape of patties from the mixture and place into the air fryer basket and cook for 8 minutes.
4. Serve and enjoy.

Healthy Salmon Patties

Preparation Time: 10 minutes

Cooking Time: 15 minutes

Serve: 4

Nutritional Value (Amount per Serving):

- Calories 60
- Fat 3.2 g
- Carbohydrates 1.9 g
- Sugar 0.5 g
- Protein 6.4 g
- Cholesterol 88 mg

Ingredients:

- 2 eggs, lightly beaten
- 2 oz salmon, cooked & flaked
- 2 tsp nutritional yeast
- 1/4 tsp paprika

- 1 tsp garlic, minced
- 1/4 cup onion, diced
- 2/3 cup almond flour
- Pepper
- Salt

Directions:

1. Preheat the air fryer to 380 F.
2. Add all ingredients into the mixing bowl and mix until well combined.
3. Make the equal shape of patties from the mixture and place into the air fryer basket and cook for 12-15 minutes.
4. Serve and enjoy.

Cheesy Salmon

Preparation Time: 10 minutes

Cooking Time: 7 minutes

Serve: 4

Nutritional Value (Amount per Serving):

- Calories 279
- Fat 14.7 g
- Carbohydrates 2.7 g
- Sugar 0.7 g
- Protein 34.6 g
- Cholesterol 81 mg

Ingredients:

- 4 salmon fillets
- 1/4 cup parmesan cheese, grated
- 3 tbsp mayonnaise

- Pepper
- Salt

Directions:

1. Preheat the air fryer to 400 F.
2. Spray air fryer basket with cooking spray.
3. In a bowl, mix cheese, mayonnaise, pepper, and salt.
4. Spread cheese mixture on top of fish fillets.
5. Place fish fillets into the air fryer basket and cook for 7 minutes.
6. Serve and enjoy.

Tasty Pesto Salmon

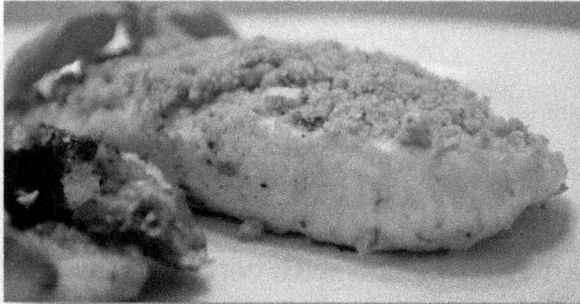

Preparation Time: 10 minutes

Cooking Time: 15 minutes

Serve: 4

Nutritional Value (Amount per Serving):

- Calories 333
- Fat 21 g
- Carbohydrates 1 g
- Sugar 1 g
- Protein 36 g
- Cholesterol 82 mg

Ingredients:

- 4 salmon fillets
- 1 tbsp olive oil
- 1/4 cup pesto

Directions:

1. Preheat the air fryer to 360 F.
2. Spray air fryer basket with cooking spray.
3. Place salmon fillets into the air fryer basket. Mix pesto and oil and spread on top of salmon fillets.
4. Cook salmon fillets for 12-15 minutes.
5. Serve and enjoy.

Everything Bagel Salmon

Preparation Time: 10 minutes

Cooking Time: 12 minutes

Serve: 2

Nutritional Value (Amount per Serving):

- Calories 355
- Fat 25 g
- Carbohydrates 0 g
- Sugar 0 g
- Protein 34.5 g
- Cholesterol 78 mg

Ingredients:

- 2 salmon fillets
- 4 tbsp everything bagel seasoning
- 2 tbsp olive oil

Directions:

1. Preheat the air fryer to 350 F.
2. Spray air fryer basket with cooking spray.
3. Brush salmon fillets with oil and coat with bagel seasoning.
4. Place fish fillets into the air fryer basket and cook for 12 minutes.
5. Serve and enjoy.

Pesto White Fish Fillets

Preparation Time: 10 minutes

Cooking Time: 8 minutes

Serve: 2

Nutritional Value (Amount per Serving):

- Calories 326
- Fat 18.6 g
- Carbohydrates 0.1 g
- Sugar 0 g
- Protein 37.8 g
- Cholesterol 119 mg

Ingredients:

- 2 white fish fillets
- 1 tbsp olive oil
- 1/4 cup basil pesto

Directions:

1. Preheat the air fryer to 360 F.
2. Spray air fryer basket with cooking spray.
3. Place fish fillets into the air fryer basket. Mix pesto and oil and spread on top of fish fillets.
4. Cook fish fillets for 8 minutes.
5. Serve and enjoy.

Bagel Crust White Fish Fillets

Preparation Time: 10 minutes

Cooking Time: 10 minutes

Serve: 4

Nutritional Value (Amount per Serving):

- Calories 281
- Fat 12.8 g
- Carbohydrates 1.2 g
- Sugar 0.2 g
- Protein 37.8 g
- Cholesterol 120 mg

Ingredients:

- 4 white fish fillets
- 1 tbsp mayonnaise
- 1 tsp lemon pepper seasoning

- 2 tbsp almond flour
- 4 tbsp everything bagel seasoning

Directions:

1. Preheat the air fryer to 375 F.
2. In a shallow dish, mix almond flour, lemon pepper seasoning, and bagel seasoning.
3. Brush fish fillets with mayonnaise and coat with almond flour mixture.
4. Place fish fillets into the air fryer basket and cook for 8-10 minutes.
5. Serve and enjoy.

Parmesan White Fish Fillets

Preparation Time: 10 minutes

Cooking Time: 15 minutes

Serve: 2

Nutritional Value (Amount per Serving):

- Calories 331
- Fat 18.7 g
- Carbohydrates 1.3 g
- Sugar 0.4 g
- Protein 38 g
- Cholesterol 119 mg

Ingredients:

- 2 white fish fillets
- 1/2 tsp paprika
- 1/2 tsp onion powder
- 1/2 tsp garlic powder

- 1/2 cup parmesan cheese, grated
- 1 tbsp olive oil
- Pepper
- Salt

Directions:

1. Preheat the air fryer to 380 F.
2. In a shallow dish, mix cheese, garlic powder, onion powder, paprika, pepper, and salt.
3. Brush fish fillets with oil and coat with cheese mixture.
4. Spray air fryer basket with cooking spray.
5. Place coated fish fillets into the air fryer basket and cook for 12-15 minutes.
6. Serve and enjoy.

Healthy Mix Vegetables

Preparation Time: 10 minutes

Cooking Time: 18 minutes

Serve: 4

Nutritional Value (Amount per Serving):

- Calories 56
- Fat 3.6 g
- Carbohydrates 5.6 g
- Sugar 2.3 g
- Protein 1.4 g
- Cholesterol 0 mg

Ingredients:

- 1 cup broccoli florets
- 1 cup carrots, sliced

- 1 cup cauliflower, cut into florets
- ¼ tsp garlic powder
- 1 tbsp olive oil
- Pepper
- Salt

Directions:

1. Add all ingredients into the bowl and toss well.
2. Add vegetable mixture into the air fryer basket and cook at 380 F for 18 minutes. Stir halfway through.
3. Serve and enjoy.

Healthy Asparagus

Preparation Time: 10 minutes

Cooking Time: 7 minutes

Serve: 4

Nutritional Value (Amount per Serving):

- Calories 35
- Fat 1.3 g
- Carbohydrates 4.4 g
- Sugar 2.1 g
- Protein 2.5 g
- Cholesterol 0 mg

Ingredients:

- 1 lb asparagus, cut the ends
- 1 tsp butter, melted
- Pepper
- Salt

Directions:

1. Preheat the air fryer to 350 F.
2. Add asparagus, butter, pepper, and salt into the bowl and toss well.
3. Add asparagus into the air fryer basket and cook for 7 minutes.
4. Serve and enjoy.

Garlic Cheese Broccoli

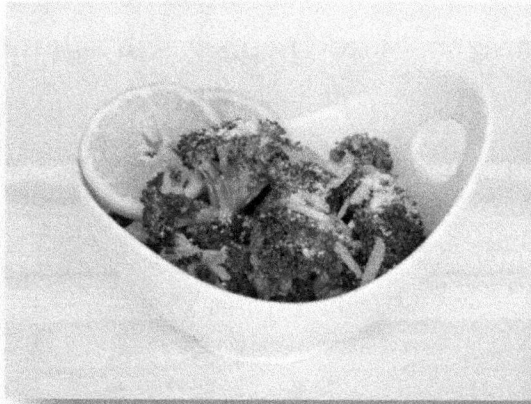

Preparation Time: 10 minutes

Cooking Time: 5 minutes

Serve: 4

Nutritional Value (Amount per Serving):

- Calories 250
- Fat 16.4 g
- Carbohydrates 8.2 g
- Sugar 2 g

- Protein 15.3 g
- Cholesterol 30 mg

Ingredients:

- 1 lb broccoli florets
- 2 tbsp butter, melted
- ¼ tsp chili flakes, crushed
- ¼ cup parmesan cheese, grated
- 1 tbsp garlic, minced
- Pepper
- Salt

Directions:

1. Preheat the air fryer to 350 F.
2. Add broccoli and remaining ingredients into the bowl and toss well.
3. Add broccoli mixture into the air fryer basket and cook for 5 minutes.
4. Serve and enjoy.

www.ingramcontent.com/pod-product-compliance
Lightning Source LLC
Chambersburg PA
CBHW050759030426
42336CB00012B/1871